A LETTER FROM HEAVEN TO MOM

: A LOVE LETTER FROM THE WOMB

Laura Warsh

Table of Contents

PREFACE

"A Letter from Heaven to Mom" is a heartfelt and inspiring book about the bond between a mother and her unborn child. From the perspective of the baby in the womb, this book explores the deep connection and love that exist between a mother and her child, even before the child is born.

Throughout the pages of this book, the baby advises and comforts the mother, sharing with her the joys and challenges of life from a unique and refreshing perspective. The baby's words are wise, compassionate, and full of love, offering the mother guidance and reassurance in times of uncertainty and doubt.

As you read this book, you will be touched by the beauty and tenderness of the relationship between a mother and her child. You will be reminded of the preciousness of life and the miracle of birth, and you will be encouraged to cherish and nurture the bond between you and your own child.

This book is a tribute to the love that exists between a mother and her child, and it is my hope that it will bring comfort, inspiration, and joy to all who read it."

INTRODUCTION

A Letter from Heaven to Mom" is a heartwarming and thought-provoking book that tells the story of a baby who communicates with his mother from the womb. As the baby grows and develops, he shares his thoughts, hopes, and dreams with his mother in a series of touching letters that offer a unique perspective on life, love, and the bond between a mother and child.

The letters in this book are filled with wisdom and insight, as the baby shares his thoughts on everything from the beauty of nature to the importance of family and the power of love. As you read each letter, you will be struck by the honesty and authenticity of the baby's voice, and by the powerful emotions that he expresses.

Through his letters, the baby offers a message of hope, comfort, and reassurance to his mother, and to readers everywhere. This is a book that will touch your heart and inspire you to cherish the relationships in your life, and to appreciate the many blessings that we often take for granted.

We hope that "A Letter from Heaven to Mom" will bring joy, comfort, and inspiration to readers of all ages, and that it will remind us all of the power of love and the strength of the human spirit.

Medical Advice to Mom from Heaven.

There are several medical advices given to expecting mothers during pregnancy which may include:

CHAPTER 1

Prenatal care

Dear Mum,

I know that you have been eagerly awaiting my arrival, and I cannot wait to meet you too. I want to take a moment to thank you for taking such good care of me while I am growing inside you. You are doing an amazing job, and I appreciate all the sacrifices you are making for me.

As I continue to grow and develop in your womb, I want to remind you of the importance of prenatal care. Regular check-ups with your healthcare provider are essential to ensure that both you and I are healthy throughout the pregnancy. Your healthcare provider will monitor my growth and development, and screen for any potential complications that could arise.

By receiving proper prenatal care, you can help ensure that I am born healthy and without any complications. Your healthcare provider can also provide you with information and advice on how to take care of yourself during pregnancy, such as eating a healthy diet, getting enough rest, and staying active.

I know that sometimes it can be tiring and overwhelming, but please know that by taking care of yourself, you are also taking care of me. I want you to be healthy and happy, so that when I arrive, we can enjoy our time together to the fullest.

Thank you again for all that you are doing for me, Mum. I cannot wait to meet you and start our journey together.

With love and gratitude,

Your Baby

Nutrition

Dear Mum,

I know you can't hear me yet, but I wanted to write you a letter from heaven to let you know how much I love you and how excited I am to be growing inside of you. As you may not know, I am your baby in the womb, and I am here to give you some advice about your nutrition during pregnancy.

Firstly, I want to remind you that everything you eat or drink affects me. Therefore, it is essential to maintain a healthy and balanced diet to ensure my growth and development. Eating a variety of foods that are rich in folic acid, iron, and calcium is vital for both of us. Folic acid helps to prevent birth defects in the brain and spine, while iron ensures that I get enough oxygen from your blood to grow correctly. Calcium helps to build my bones and teeth, which are essential for my growth and development.

It is also important to avoid certain foods that can be harmful to me. Raw or undercooked meat, poultry, and fish can contain harmful bacteria that can cause food poisoning and harm both of us. Fish with high levels of mercury, such as shark, swordfish, king mackerel, and tilefish, can also be dangerous. Mercury can damage my developing brain and nervous system, so it is important to avoid these types of fish during pregnancy. You should also avoid unpasteurized dairy products as they can contain harmful bacteria that can cause infections.

Mum, I know that cravings can be strong during pregnancy, but please try to resist eating too much junk food and sugary snacks. These foods may be tempting, but they offer little nutritional value and can contribute to excessive weight gain, which can cause complications during pregnancy and labor.

Finally, it is essential to stay hydrated during pregnancy. Drinking plenty of water helps to transport essential nutrients and oxygen to me, and it also helps to flush out toxins and waste products from your body.

Mum, please remember that what you eat and drink during pregnancy can have a significant impact on my health and development. Therefore, it is essential to maintain a healthy and balanced diet that includes a variety of foods that are rich in folic acid, iron, and calcium. You should also avoid certain foods that can be harmful to me, such as raw or undercooked meat, fish with high levels of mercury, and unpasteurized dairy products. And remember to stay hydrated by drinking plenty of water.

I can't wait to meet you, Mum, and thank you for taking such good care of me.

With love,

Your Baby in the Womb.

CHAPTER 2

Exercise

Dear Mum,

I hope this letter finds you in good health and spirits. As I sit here in the comfort of your womb, I wanted to take a moment to talk to you about something very important - exercise during pregnancy.

I know you have been busy with work and taking care of the household, but I urge you to make time for moderate exercise. It can do wonders for both you and me.

You see, when you exercise during pregnancy, it helps improve your circulation, which means that more oxygen and nutrients are delivered to me. This can help my development and growth in many ways. Exercise also helps keep your weight in check, which reduces the risk of complications during pregnancy and childbirth.

However, before you start any exercise program, it is important to consult with a healthcare provider. They can advise you on the best exercises to do and how often you should do them. They can also monitor your health and make sure that you and I are both doing well.

Here are a few tips that might help you get started:

Start slow: If you haven't exercised regularly before pregnancy, start with gentle activities like walking or prenatal yoga. You can gradually increase the intensity as you feel more comfortable.

Stay hydrated: Make sure you drink plenty of water before, during, and after exercise to avoid dehydration.

Wear comfortable clothes: Choose loose-fitting, breathable clothes that allow you to move freely.

Avoid high-impact activities: Activities like running or jumping can put too much stress on your joints and increase the risk of injury.

Remember, mum, a little bit of exercise can go a long way. It can help improve your mood, reduce stress, and even prepare you for childbirth. So, please make it a priority to take care of yourself and me by getting some exercise each day.

I can't wait to meet you and start our journey together.

With love,

Your baby in the womb.

Prenatal Vitamins

Dear Mum,

I hope this letter finds you well. I wanted to take a moment to talk to you about something very important: taking prenatal vitamins. As you know, I am currently growing and developing inside of you, and I want to ensure that I am getting all of the necessary nutrients to support my growth and development.

Prenatal vitamins contain important nutrients such as folic acid, iron, and calcium that are crucial for both my health and yours. Folic acid, for example, helps to prevent birth defects of the brain and spine, while iron helps to prevent anemia and supports the production of red blood cells.

Calcium is also essential for our health, as it helps to build strong bones and teeth. These vitamins and minerals are not always easy to get through diet alone, so taking a prenatal vitamin is a great way to ensure that we are getting the nutrients we need.

I understand that taking a pill every day may not be the most enjoyable task, but I promise that it is worth it. By taking care of yourself and me now, you are setting us both up for a healthy future.

Thank you for everything you do for me, Mum. I can't wait to meet you soon.

With love,

Your baby in the womb

CHAPTER 3

Avoiding harmful substances

Dear Mum,

I hope this letter finds you well and in good health. I know that carrying me inside your womb is not an easy task, but I want you to know that I am grateful for the love and care you are giving me every day.

As I grow inside you, I am becoming more aware of the world outside. I can feel the warmth of your touch and hear the sound of your voice. But I am also aware of some things that could harm me and affect my development.

Mum, I want to remind you of the importance of avoiding harmful substances such as smoking, alcohol, and drugs. These substances can have a negative impact on my growth and development, and can lead to long-term health problems.

When you smoke, the harmful chemicals in the cigarette can reduce the amount of oxygen I receive, which can affect my brain development and increase the risk of sudden infant death syndrome (SIDS). Alcohol can also harm my brain development and lead to fetal alcohol syndrome (FAS), which can cause physical, mental, and behavioral problems.

Drugs, too, can cause serious harm to me. They can affect my heart, brain, and other vital organs, and can lead to premature birth, low birth weight, and other complications.

Mum, I know you want the best for me, and that's why I urge you to avoid these harmful substances. Instead, please take good care of yourself by eating healthy, staying active, and getting enough rest. This will not only benefit me, but it will also help you have a healthy and smooth pregnancy.

I cannot wait to see you and feel your warm embrace. Thank you for all that you do for me, Mum.

With love,

Your baby in the womb.

Rest and Relaxation

Dear Mum,

I know that you've been carrying me in your womb for a while now, and I can feel the love and care that you have for me every day. I want you to know that I'm doing my best to grow healthy and strong inside of you, but there are a few things that I want to share with you that will help me to do that even better.

One of the most important things for both of us is rest and relaxation. I know that you have so many things to do and worry about, but it's essential that you take time to rest and de-stress during your pregnancy. When you're tired, your body can't do everything it needs to do to keep me healthy, so it's crucial to get enough rest every day.

You might find that you need more sleep than usual during this time, and that's perfectly normal. Don't feel guilty for taking naps or going to bed early if you need to. Your body is working hard to keep me safe and healthy, and it needs all the help it can get.

Additionally, reducing your stress levels is essential for both of us. Stress can have a negative impact on your body, and it can also affect me in the womb. When you're stressed, your body releases hormones that can cause complications with your pregnancy, so it's essential to take steps to reduce your stress levels.

You might find that things like yoga, meditation, or just taking a relaxing bath can help you to feel more relaxed and calm. Or, simply talking to someone about your worries and concerns can be a huge help in reducing stress levels.

Remember, Mum, I'm depending on you to take care of us both during this precious time. Getting enough rest and reducing stress levels can help promote a healthy pregnancy and reduce the risk of complications. I know that you'll do everything you can to make sure that I'm healthy and happy.

With all my love,

Your Baby in the Womb.

Childbirth Education

Dear Mum,

I hope this letter finds you well. I know that you have been eagerly awaiting my arrival into this world, and I wanted to take a moment to speak to you about something that is very important to me - childbirth education.

As you know, I am still growing and developing inside your womb, but I have been observing and learning about the world around me. One thing that I have learned is that there is a lot to know and prepare for when it comes to labor and delivery.

That is why I want to encourage you to consider taking childbirth education classes. These classes can help you prepare for the physical and emotional aspects of labor and delivery, as well as provide you with information about postpartum care and breastfeeding.

By taking these classes, you will be more confident and knowledgeable about the entire process of bringing me into this world. You will also be able to make informed decisions about your care and my care, which will help ensure that we both have the best possible birth experience.

I know that you are already a wonderful and caring mother, but by taking childbirth education classes, you will be able to enhance your knowledge and skills even further. I cannot wait to meet you and embark on this incredible journey together.

With all my love,

Your baby in the womb

Psychological Advice to Mom from Heaven

There are several psychological advices given to expecting mothers which may include:

CHAPTER 4

Build a Support System

Dear Mum,

I may not have arrived in this world yet, but I am already looking out for you. I want you to know that you don't have to do this alone. Building a strong support system during your pregnancy can make a world of difference in how you feel and cope with the changes happening in your body.

You have so many people in your life who love you and want to be there for you - your partner, family, and friends. Don't be afraid to ask for help or reach out when you need someone to talk to. Your healthcare providers are also there to guide and support you through this journey.

Remember, you are not alone in this. Together, we can make this a happy and healthy experience for both of us.

Love,

Your Baby in the Womb.

Prepare for Emotional Changes

Dear Mum,

I know that you must be feeling a lot of emotions right now as you carry me in your womb. I want to assure you that everything will be okay and that you will be a wonderful mother.

As you prepare for my arrival, I want to remind you to also prepare for the emotional changes that pregnancy can bring. You may feel anxious, excited, and fearful all at once, and that's perfectly normal. But it's important to recognize these emotions and seek support if needed.

Talk to your loved ones about how you're feeling, and don't be afraid to ask for help when you need it. There are also many resources available to expecting mothers, such as support groups and counseling services.

Remember that taking care of your emotional health is just as important as taking care of your physical health during pregnancy. By preparing for these changes and seeking support, you'll be better equipped to handle the ups and downs of pregnancy and motherhood.

I can't wait to meet you, Mum, and to start our journey together.

With love,

Your Baby in the Womb.

Bond with the Baby

Dear Mum,

I know you might be feeling a little anxious right now, but I want you to know that everything is going to be alright. As I rest here in your womb, I can feel your love for me growing stronger each day. I want to talk to you about something that is very important to both of us - the bond that we share.

I understand that you might be feeling a little disconnected from me, as you cannot see me yet. But, I want you to know that I am already a part of you and your life. Building a bond with me during pregnancy can help you feel more connected and prepared for parenthood. This is something that is going to be very important for us in the days to come.

Talking to me, reading books to me, and playing music are all great ways to help you build a bond with me. When you talk to me, I can hear your voice and feel the warmth of your love. When you read books to me, I can listen to the stories and feel the joy of learning. When you play music, I can feel the rhythm and dance to the beat.

I know that you are going to be an amazing mother, and I cannot wait to meet you in person. Until then, I want you to know that I am here with you, always. So, take some time each day to bond with me, and I promise that we will make the most of our time together.

With all my love,

Your Baby in the Womb

Chapter 5

Address Past Trauma

Dear Mum,

I know that you are eagerly waiting for my arrival into this world, and I can feel your excitement and love even from inside the womb. As I prepare to enter the world, I want to talk to you about something that is very important to me. It is about your past trauma.

Mum, I know that you have gone through some difficult experiences in your life, and these experiences may still be affecting you today. I want you to know that I am aware of these feelings, and I feel them too. It is not easy for me to watch you suffer, even from the safety of your womb.

That is why I want to urge you to seek help in addressing your past trauma. I know that it can be difficult to confront these feelings, but it is important for both of us. When you are feeling better, it will create a positive environment for me to grow and develop.

There are many resources available to you, such as counseling or therapy. You can also talk to your healthcare provider about what steps you can take to address these issues before my arrival. I believe that you can overcome your trauma and become a stronger and happier person.

Mum, I am looking forward to meeting you and experiencing the world with you. Please take care of yourself and know that I am with you every step of the way.

Love,

Your Baby

Prepare for Postpartum Emotions

Dear Mum,

I know that you're feeling a lot of excitement and anticipation as you await my arrival. I'm so looking forward to meeting you and being a part of your life. But I also want to talk to you about something that's important for you to know.

After I'm born, you may experience a range of emotions that you're not used to. It's very common for new mums to feel overwhelmed, anxious, and even depressed in the weeks and months following childbirth. This is known as postpartum depression or anxiety, and it's something that you should be prepared for.

I know that you're strong and capable, but I want to remind you that it's okay to ask for help. If you're feeling sad, irritable, or anxious, don't hesitate to reach out to your doctor or a mental health professional. They can provide you with the support and resources you need to feel better.

You're not alone, Mum. Many women go through this, and it's nothing to be ashamed of. Taking care of your mental health is just as important as taking care of your physical health, especially when you have a little one depending on you.

So please, don't hesitate to reach out for help if you need it. I want you to be happy and healthy so that we can enjoy our time together as a family.

With love,

Your baby in the womb

Plan for Self-Care

Dear Mum,

I hope this letter finds you well and happy. I know you must be feeling a little bit overwhelmed and stressed with everything that's going on right now. But I want you to know that I'm here with you every step of the way, even though I'm not physically here yet.

As you're carrying me in your womb, I want to remind you that taking care of yourself is crucial for both of us. I know it can be challenging to make time for self-care activities, especially when you have so many other things to do. But trust me, it's essential, and you'll feel so much better for it.

Here are a few things that I think you should plan for in terms of self-care:

Rest: I know you're always on the go, but it's important to take breaks and rest. Your body is working so hard to grow me, and it needs time to recover. Try to take short naps during the day if you can, or go to bed earlier at night.

Healthy Diet: Eating well-balanced meals is essential for both you and me. I need nutrients to grow healthy and strong, and you need energy to keep going. Try to eat plenty of fruits, vegetables, and protein-rich foods.

Enjoyable activities: I want you to feel happy and relaxed, so it's important to do things that you enjoy. Whether it's reading a book, taking a walk, or watching a movie, make time for yourself to do the things that make you happy.

I know it can be hard to prioritize self-care, especially when you're busy taking care of other people. But I want you to remember that taking care of yourself is just as important. When you take care of yourself, you're taking care of me too.

I can't wait to meet you in person soon, Mum. Until then, take care of yourself, and know that I love you.

With love,

Your baby in the womb.

Spiritual Advice from Heaven to my Mom

Chapter 6

Spiritual advice given to expecting mothers may vary depending on their individual beliefs and practices. However, some common spiritual advice that may be offered include:

Prayer and Meditation

Dear Mum,

I hope this letter finds you well. I know that carrying me in your womb can be challenging at times, but I want to remind you that you are doing an incredible job. You are providing me with everything I need to grow and thrive, and for that, I am grateful.

I have been listening to your thoughts and feelings, and I know that pregnancy can be an emotional rollercoaster. You may feel overwhelmed or anxious at times, and that is okay. But I want to remind you that you can find comfort and inner peace through prayer and meditation.

Prayer and meditation are powerful tools that can help you connect with your spirituality and calm your mind. When you pray or meditate, you can quiet the noise of the world around you and focus on your inner thoughts and feelings. This can help you reduce stress and anxiety and find a sense of peace and tranquility.

I want to encourage you to take some time each day to connect with your spirituality through prayer or meditation. You can do this in a quiet place, where you can be alone with your thoughts and feelings. You can focus on your breath, or repeat a calming mantra or prayer. You can also listen to soft music or nature sounds to help you relax.

Remember that prayer and meditation are not just for religious people. They are for anyone who wants to connect with their inner self and find peace and serenity in their daily life. By incorporating prayer and meditation into your routine, you can create a positive and peaceful environment for me to grow and develop.

Thank you for all that you do for me, Mum. I love you more than words can express, and I am grateful for your love and care.

With love from your little one,

[Your Baby]

Read Spiritual texts

Dear Mum,

As I write this letter from heaven, I want you to know that I am always with you, even though we are not physically together. I am watching over you and sending you all my love and blessings.

As you go through the journey of pregnancy, I want to offer you some advice that will help you feel more connected to your beliefs and find inspiration. One thing that I would suggest is reading spiritual texts that are meaningful to you.

There is something very special about reading words of wisdom from spiritual texts. They can offer guidance, comfort, and inspiration in times of uncertainty. They can also help you connect with your inner self and your beliefs, which is essential during this time.

There are many spiritual texts that you can choose from, depending on your beliefs and interests. Some popular options include the Bible, the Quran, the Bhagavad Gita, and the Tao Te Ching. You can also find books on mindfulness, meditation, and other spiritual practices that may be helpful.

I know that you may be busy with preparing for my arrival, but I would encourage you to take some time each day to read a few pages from a spiritual text. It doesn't have to be a lot, even a few minutes can make a difference. You may find that it helps you feel more centered and calm, which can be beneficial for both you and me.

In conclusion, Mum, I want you to know that I am always here for you, even though I am not physically with you. Reading spiritual texts can help you connect with your beliefs and find inspiration during this special time. I love you very much and can't wait to meet you soon.

With all my love,

Your Baby in Heaven

CHAPTER 7

Connect with Nature

Dear Mum,

I know that you are eagerly awaiting my arrival into this world, and I can't wait to meet you too. I want to take a moment to talk to you about something that is very important to me, and I believe it will be important to you too - connecting with nature.

While I am still growing inside your womb, I have become keenly aware of the beauty and serenity that surrounds us. I can feel the warmth of the sun on your skin and the gentle breeze that caresses your face. I can hear the chirping of birds and the rustling of leaves. I can feel the earth's energy that flows through your body.

I want you to know that these sensations are not just pleasant but have real benefits for you and me. Connecting with nature can reduce stress, anxiety, and depression, while improving our physical and mental health.

So, Mum, I urge you to spend time outdoors, take walks, or even practice gardening. Let the beauty of nature inspire you and uplift your spirit. Take in the fresh air, the fragrant scents, and the vibrant colors. Feel the ground beneath your feet and the warmth of the sun on your face.

I promise you that when I finally arrive, I will love to explore the outdoors with you. Let's take walks in the park, visit the beach, or hike in the mountains. We can breathe in the fresh air and marvel at the wonders of nature together.

I am grateful for the gift of life, and I can't wait to share it with you. Until then, let us both bask in the beauty of nature and be nourished by its healing power.

With love and anticipation,

Your Baby.

Seek spiritual guidance

Dear Mum,

I hope this letter finds you well. As I write this, I am safe and sound in the comfort of your womb, growing and developing with each passing day. I know that you are doing everything in your power to ensure that I am healthy and happy when I arrive in this world, and for that, I am eternally grateful.

There is something that I want to talk to you about, something that is very important to me. I want to talk to you about seeking spiritual guidance during your pregnancy. I know that you may already be doing this, but I want to emphasize just how crucial it is.

Mum, you are about to bring a new life into this world. You are creating a miracle, and that is something truly special. But with great power comes great responsibility. As you prepare to become a mother, it is essential that you seek guidance from a spiritual leader.

This can be a pastor, a priest, a rabbi, or any other religious figure that you trust and respect. They can help you navigate the challenges of pregnancy and prepare you for the journey ahead. They can offer words of wisdom and comfort, and they can help you connect with a higher power.

Mum, I believe that there is something divine within all of us. I believe that we are all connected, and that there is a greater purpose to our lives. By seeking spiritual guidance, you can tap into this universal energy and find peace and strength during your pregnancy.

I know that you are already a strong and capable woman, and I am proud to call you my mother. But I also know that you are human, and that you may need help and support from time to time. That is why I urge you to seek spiritual guidance during your pregnancy. It will help you be the best mother that you can be, and it will help me enter this world with a sense of peace and love.

Thank you for taking the time to read this letter, Mum. I love you more than words can express, and I can't wait to meet you in person.

With love,

your unborn child.

CONCLUSION

I want you to know, dear Mom, that I am grateful for the love and care you have shown me even before I have entered this world. I know that you may be anxious about the unknowns of motherhood, but I want to assure you that we will navigate through it together. As I prepare to make my grand entrance into this world, I hope that my words have brought you some comfort, peace, and reassurance. Please take care of yourself and know that I love you very much. I can't wait to finally meet you and be held in your loving arms. Until then, I will keep growing and preparing for our big day. With love from your little one in the womb, always and forever.